INSULIN INDEPENDENCE

Holistic Therapies For Type 1 Diabetes Management

Explore Holistic Approaches To Manage Type 1 Diabetes And Reduce Reliance On Insulin Through Innovative Therapies

DR. BRIDGET PROMISE

Table of Contents

CHAPTER ONE

Introduction

Type 1 diabetes is a chronic medical condition distinguished by the body's incapacity to synthesize insulin, an essential hormone for the regulation of blood glucose levels.

In contrast to type 2 diabetes, which is frequently correlated with lifestyle choices, type 1 diabetes is classified as an autoimmune disorder due to the erroneous targeting and destruction of pancreatic cells responsible for producing insulin by the immune system. Survival-threatening complications of this condition require permanent reliance on insulin injections or an insulin device. In recent times, there has been an increasing inclination towards investigating methods to attain insulin independence and embracing holistic strategies for the more efficient management of type 1 diabetes.

Comprehension Of Type 1 Diabetes

To fully grasp the importance of exploring alternatives to insulin reliance, it is critical to immerse oneself in the foundational principles of type 1 diabetes. Positioned posterior to the stomach, the pancreas is an essential organ that regulates blood sugar levels. Type 1 diabetes is characterized by an immune response that targets insulin-producing beta cells in the pancreas, mistaking them for foreign pathogens. This results in the elimination of these beta cells. As a result, the body's capacity to generate insulin is compromised.

Insulin plays a vital role in facilitating the transportation of glucose into cells, thereby supplying them with the energy required for optimal operation. Glucose accumulates in the circulation in the absence of adequate insulin, resulting in elevated blood sugar levels. Neglecting to address this condition may lead to severe complications including cardiovascular disease, renal impairment, and neuropathy.

Historically, exogenous insulin administration, whether via injections or an insulin device, has been the cornerstone of type 1 diabetes management. This approach aims to replicate the functionality of the body's endogenous insulin secretion.

The Struggle For Independence From Insulin

Exogenous insulin continues to be an indispensable life-sustaining intervention for individuals diagnosed with type 1 diabetes; however, the pursuit of insulin independence has persisted. Scholars and medical practitioners have been investigating novel methodologies to either rectify the impairment of beta cells or identify substitute mechanisms for blood sugar regulation that do not exclusively depend on insulin injections.

Beta cell transplantation is an auspicious pathway in the pursuit of insulin independence. By implantation of insulin-producing cells into the pancreas, this procedure attempts to restore the body's natural insulin production capacity. Nevertheless, substantial barriers remain, including the limited availability of donor cells and the requirement for immunosuppressive medications to avert rejection.

An alternative methodology entails the generation of insulin-producing cells via stem cell technology. Stem cell therapy possesses the capacity to reinstate adequate insulin production by substituting impaired beta cells. Although this area of study is still in its nascent phase, it presents a glimmer of optimism regarding the possibility that in the future, people with type 1 diabetes might not be exclusively reliant on exogenous insulin sources.

CHAPTER TWO

A Holistic Approach To The Management Of Type 1 Diabetes

Apart from the endeavor to achieve insulin independence, an increasing number of individuals are acknowledging the significance of implementing a comprehensive strategy for the management of type 1 diabetes.

In addition to insulin therapy, the integration of lifestyle adjustments, dietary selections, and complementary therapies can significantly contribute to the enhancement of general health and regulation of blood sugar.

Tailored nutrition is a critical component of holistic diabetes management. Implementing a personalized and well-balanced dietary regimen can effectively manage blood glucose levels and diminish the need for insulin.

An alimentation abundant in unprocessed carbohydrates, fiber-rich, and deficient in refined sugars may aid in the regulation of blood sugar. Moreover, certain individuals diagnosed with type 1 diabetes discover beneficial outcomes by implementing low-carbohydrate or ketogenic diets, which aid in the regulation of blood glucose levels.

Consistent physical activity constitutes an additional crucial element of comprehensive diabetes management. Physical activity not only aids in the regulation of body weight but also improves the body's sensitivity to insulin, thereby enabling more efficient utilization of the hormone.

A combination of strength training, flexibility exercises, and aerobic exercise can positively affect blood sugar regulation and overall health.

Management of stress is an integral component of comprehensive diabetes care. Because chronic stress can cause an increase in blood sugar levels, individuals with type 1 diabetes must integrate daily mindfulness, yoga, meditation, or other stress-reducing practices. Inadequate sleep can disrupt metabolic health and blood sugar levels, making adequate sleep an additional necessity.

Complementary therapies, including herbal supplements and

acupuncture, are gaining prominence in the field of holistic diabetes management. Although these methods may not serve as substitutes for insulin therapy, certain individuals may discover that they enhance conventional treatments and promote holistic health.

It is imperative to acknowledge that the holistic approach to managing type 1 diabetes is exceedingly personalized. What is effective for one individual might not apply to another. Hence, continuous cooperation with healthcare experts is imperative to customize a comprehensive care strategy that attends to the distinct requirements and inclinations of every patient.

Type 1 diabetes poses an enduring obstacle, necessitating consistent monitoring of blood glucose levels and administration of insulin daily.

Although insulin continues to be an essential component of treatment, the pursuit of insulin independence and the implementation of holistic approaches provide optimism for those afflicted with type 1 diabetes in terms of improved quality of life. Promising developments in the field of medical research, including stem cell therapy and beta cell transplantation, may one day enable people to experience a diminished dependence on external insulin sources.

Personalized nutrition, consistent engagement in physical activity, effective stress management, and complementary therapies are all crucial components in the comprehensive management of diabetes. Acknowledging the individuality of each person's experience with type 1 diabetes, the primary focus is on customizing an all-encompassing care strategy that attends to the physical, mental, and emotional dimensions of health. Using continuous research and a dedication to personalized attention, the management of type 1 diabetes is ever more dynamic, presenting individuals with this condition with fresh opportunities and pathways.

Striking A Balance Between Nutrition And Diet

Attaining optimal health is a complex undertaking encompassing numerous interrelated components, with the fundamental notion of achieving a harmonious equilibrium between diet and nutrition serving as its foundation. The dietary choices we make have a profound impact on our general health, regulating vital signs such as energy levels and the prevention of diseases. Ensuring an optimal equilibrium between diet and nutrition is of paramount importance in sustaining a healthy lifestyle and averting an extensive array of health complications, such as diabetes.

An optimal diet comprises a variety of essential nutrients, such as carbohydrates, proteins, lipids, vitamins, and minerals. Proteins aid in muscle repair and development, whereas carbohydrates serve as the principal source of energy. Several physiological processes, including hormone synthesis and nutrient assimilation, rely on fats, which are frequently misconstrued. By serving as catalysts for a multitude of biochemical reactions, vitamins and minerals promote bone health and immune function, among other things.

In the case of individuals who are managing diabetes, it is even more imperative to adhere to a balanced diet. It is essential to closely monitor carbohydrate consumption, as carbohydrates have a direct impact on blood glucose levels. Consuming a diet abundant in healthy lipids, whole cereals, fiber, and lean proteins can aid in blood sugar regulation and promote overall health. A second crucial element is portion control, which ensures that caloric expenditure corresponds with energy consumption to prevent complications associated with weight gain, which is a prevalent issue among people with diabetes.

Physical Activity and Well-Being:

Engaging in physical activity is fundamental to maintaining a healthy lifestyle and is instrumental in the prevention and management of diabetes. Consistent physical activity provides an extensive array of advantages, such as enhanced insulin sensitivity, improved weight management, and improved cardiovascular health. Physical well-being and exercise are inextricably linked, with each factor influencing and strengthening the other in a perpetual cycle of favorable consequences.

By enhancing insulin sensitivity, aerobic exercises such as brisk walking, jogging, and cycling help regulate blood sugar levels. In contrast, strength training activities promote muscle growth, thereby facilitating glucose metabolism and enhancing metabolic health as a whole. In addition, consistent engagement in physical activity aids in the regulation of body weight, thereby mitigating the likelihood of complications commonly linked to diabetes and obesity.

In addition to its physical advantages, exercise has a beneficial effect on one's mental health. Participating in physical activity stimulates the secretion of endorphins, which are neurotransmitters that elicit emotions of joy and alleviate anxiety. Because stress hormones can cause an increase in blood sugar, individuals with diabetes must pay special attention to stress management.

By integrating practices such as yoga or meditation into a daily exercise regimen, one can cultivate a comprehensive perspective on wellness that encompasses the physical and mental dimensions.

CHAPTER THREE
Connecting The Mind And Body In Diabetes Management

The interplay between the mind and body is a complex and profound relationship that has a substantial impact on the management of diabetes. The interrelation between mental health, emotional state, and tension has been extensively studied about physical health.

It is vital for individuals managing the complexities of diabetes to comprehend this interdependence.

Blood sugar levels can be substantially impacted by stress in particular. The human body reacts to physical or emotional tension by secreting stress hormones such as cortisol and adrenaline. The potential consequence of these hormones is an elevation in blood glucose levels, which can pose a difficulty for those who have diabetes.

The incorporation of relaxation techniques, mindfulness practices, or participation in pastimes has the potential to exert a positive impact on the management of diabetes.

Furthermore, the influence of emotions and mental health on lifestyle decisions, such as medication adherence and dietary patterns, should not be overlooked. It is imperative to consider and manage any underlying psychological factors, including anxiety or depression, to provide overall diabetes care. Developing a robust support network, comprising family members, friends, healthcare practitioners, and medical personnel, can significantly improve one's emotional health and coping mechanisms when confronted with the difficulties associated with diabetes.

Investigating Complementary Therapies

In the realm of diabetes management, the investigation of alternative therapies has become increasingly prominent as the healthcare industry evolves. Although conventional medical methods continue to be essential, alternative therapies provide supplementary pathways to improve overall health and approach the management of diabetes more holistically.

Acupuncture is one such alternative therapy that is gaining popularity. Acupuncture, which has its origins in traditional Chinese medicine, stimulates energy flow through the implantation of thin needles into specific sites on the body.

Acupuncture may increase insulin sensitivity and alleviate diabetes-related symptoms, according to several studies. Nevertheless, patients and physicians alike who are contemplating alternative therapies must communicate to ascertain whether or not they are compatible with their comprehensive treatment regimen.

An additional area of inquiry pertains to medicinal supplements. Research has been conducted on specific botanicals, including fenugreek and bitter melon, to determine their potential efficacy in the management of diabetes. Potential benefits of these botanicals include reduced blood sugar and enhanced insulin sensitivity.

Nevertheless, similar to any dietary supplement, herbal therapies should be utilized with extreme caution and under the supervision of healthcare professionals, due to the possibility of drug interactions and unintended adverse effects.

Mind-body techniques, such as guided imagery, biofeedback, and meditation, also provide alternative methods for managing diabetes. These methods emphasize the utilization of mental capabilities to influence physical health positively. Incorporating mindfulness practices into one's daily existence may benefit blood sugar regulation and overall health, according to research.

In summary, integrated components of a holistic approach to diabetes management include attaining a state of equilibrium in one's diet and nutrition, engaging in consistent physical activity, acknowledging the correlation between the mind and body, and investigating alternative therapeutic modalities. Every constituent in its way contributes distinctively to the complex fabric of wellness, providing individuals with diabetes with the resources and understanding necessary to lead satisfying and sound lives. Patients must collaborate closely with their healthcare providers to customize these strategies to their particular requirements, thereby guaranteeing an effective and individualized diabetes management regimen.

Herbal Supplements And Nutraceuticals: A Holistic Approach To Health

There is a growing trend among individuals to incorporate nutraceuticals and botanical supplements into their wellness regimens to achieve optimal health. Natural remedies, which are obtained from dietary sources and are said to have health benefits, provide a comprehensive approach to the preservation of overall wellness. Combining the terms "nutrition" and "pharmaceuticals," nutraceuticals comprise an extensive array of substances, such as medicinal extracts, vitamins, minerals, and dietary supplements. Within this particular framework, we investigate the potential of herbal supplements and nutraceuticals to address distinct health issues, including but not limited to sleep disturbances, mental well-being, and blood sugar regulation.

A Nutraceutical Approach to Stress Management and Mental Health

It is widely acknowledged that stress negatively impacts mental health and has become an unavoidable component of contemporary life. Nutraceuticals are of paramount importance in the realm of stress management and the enhancement of mental health. The increasing prevalence of adaptogenic botanicals such as rhodiola and ashwagandha is due to their stress-relieving properties. It is hypothesized that by assisting the body in adjusting to stressors, these botanicals can mitigate the physiological and psychological effects of chronic stress.

Fish oil-derived omega-3 fatty acids, which are dietary supplements, have demonstrated potential in promoting mental health. Critical to the operation of the brain, these fatty acids may aid in the alleviation of symptoms related to depression and anxiety. In addition, chamomile and valerian root-infused botanical beverages are renowned for their soothing properties, which aid in tension reduction and relaxation.

The Effects of Sleep on Blood Sugar: Investigating Natural Remedies

The complex correlation between sleep patterns and glycemic levels has received heightened interest in recent times. Deficiencies in sleep quality or quantity, which are inadequate, may contribute to the development of insulin resistance and subsequently result in hyperglycemia. Herbal supplements and nutraceuticals present potential remedies for enhancing sleep quality and reducing its adverse effects on blood sugar levels.

Supplementary melatonin, an endogenous hormone responsible for regulating sleep-wake cycles, has been associated with enhanced sleep quality. Sedative properties are also associated with herbal remedies such as valerian root and passionflower, which promote relaxation and facilitate a more restful night's slumber.

Furthermore, magnesium, an essential mineral present in a variety of grains, seeds, and verdant greens, is implicated in the regulation of sleep. Magnesium supplementation may enhance the quality of sleep for those who are deficient in this mineral.

CHAPTER FOUR

Technology In Diabetes Management: Nutraceutical Integration

The prevalence of technology integration in diabetes management has witnessed a notable increase in tandem with its ongoing advancements. Nutraceuticals serve a supplementary function within this framework, providing adjunctive remedies to traditional approaches to managing diabetes.

An exemplary instance pertains to the application of cinnamon as a nutraceutical supplement in the treatment of diabetes. Research findings indicate that cinnamon might exert a beneficial influence on blood glucose levels, thereby establishing its potential utility as a dietary supplement for individuals coping with diabetes. Nevertheless, individuals must consult with healthcare professionals to ascertain the optimal dosage and verify potential drug interactions.

About technology-assisted diabetes management, monitoring blood sugar levels, dietary consumption, and physical activity is facilitated via wearable devices and mobile applications.

Incorporating nutraceuticals into diabetes-friendly diets can function as a natural supplement to these technologies.

In Conclusion, The Adoption Of A Balanced Lifestyle

Within the dynamic realm of health and wellness, nutraceuticals and botanical supplements present individuals with a means to attain comprehensive and balanced wellness. Using stress management, mental health promotion, sleep improvement, and diabetes management supplementation, these all-natural remedies offer beneficial instruments for individuals in pursuit of a holistic and well-rounded approach to health.

Nonetheless, individuals must exercise utmost caution when considering the utilization of nutraceuticals. It is imperative to seek guidance from healthcare professionals, comprehend the unique health requirements of each individual, and incorporate these supplements into a more comprehensive lifestyle approach to fully capitalize on their potential advantages. With the proliferation of natural remedies, technological advancements, and scientific convergence, individuals are presented with the prospect of adopting a holistic and individualized health approach that incorporates conventional and contemporary remedies.

Tailored Treatment Strategies

Type 1 diabetes is an especially intricate and challenging chronic condition that necessitates an individualized strategy for control.

There is a growing trend away from the one-size-fits-all treatment model towards customized approaches that take into account individual variances, lifestyle components, and the distinct obstacles encountered by each person. This investigation examines personalized treatment plans for Type 1 diabetes, focusing on the complexities of managing the condition.

It analyzes concrete case studies of individuals who have successfully achieved insulin independence, underscores the significance of establishing a supportive lifestyle, stresses the importance of collaborating with healthcare professionals, and offers prospects for diabetes management.

CHAPTER FIVE

Case Studies: Actual Accounts Of Self-Sufficiency In Insulin

Achieving insulin independence is an aspiration shared by numerous individuals diagnosed with Type 1 diabetes. Although not universally achievable, notable advances in personalized treatment plans have facilitated noteworthy instances of success. The aforementioned case studies offer valuable insights into the experiences of individuals who, using meticulously designed and individualized strategies, were able to diminish or eradicate their reliance on insulin.

Sarah, a 35-year-old individual who was diagnosed with Type 1 diabetes when she was 12 years old, is one such case. By integrating continuous glucose monitoring (CGM), tailored dietary modifications, and an individualized exercise regimen, Sarah achieved a substantial reduction in her insulin needs. As time passed, her adherence to an individualized treatment regimen resulted in phases of self-sustenance from insulin, demonstrating the efficacy of customized approaches in the realm of diabetes control.

Establishing A Nurturing Way Of Life

Personalized treatment programs transcend the use of insulin and medication regimens. The management of diabetes is significantly influenced by one's lifestyle, and embracing a supportive way of life can have a positive effect on one's overall health. Particularly in regards to stress management, dietary habits, and physical activity, individuals diagnosed with Type 1 diabetes are realizing the significance of customizing their way of life to suit their particular requirements.

As an illustration, Mark, a professional aged 28 years, discovered that the integration of consistent mindfulness exercises into his daily regimen facilitated the regulation of his stress levels, ultimately resulting in improved glycemic control. Constructing a supportive lifestyle necessitates the identification of personal triggers, be they associated with physical activity, nutrition, or psychological welfare, and the formulation of deliberate decisions to alleviate their influence on the management of diabetes.

Partnership With Healthcare Specialists

Achieving personalized treatment plans necessitates the active participation and cooperation of healthcare professionals and individuals diagnosed with Type 1 diabetes. The conventional paradigm of a physician prescribing a standard treatment regimen is transforming into a collaborative alliance in which patients participate actively in the decision-making process. This collaborative methodology acknowledges the distinctive elements of diabetes management for every individual and guarantees that treatment strategies are according to their objectives and way of life.

Emma, a Type 1 diabetic who is 42 years old, stresses the value of maintaining transparent lines of communication with her healthcare team. Ongoing consultations, the exchange of knowledge derived from continuous glucose monitoring, and the modification of treatment strategies by real-time data have been integral components in Emma's pursuit of individualized healthcare. This collaboration cultivates a feeling of empowerment among individuals with Type 1 diabetes, as they are actively engaged in the process of formulating their treatment plans.

Prospects for the Future of Type 1 Diabetes Management

As technological progress persists, the outlook for the management of type 1 diabetes appears auspicious. A convergence of artificial intelligence, precision medicine, and wearable devices is reshaping the therapeutic landscape. Smart algorithms, continuous glucose monitors, and insulin pumps are increasingly recognized as essential elements in the management of diabetes. These devices offer personalized insights and real-time data.

There is hope that in the future, closed-loop systems will be even more sophisticated, allowing devices to modify insulin delivery autonomously in response to glucose levels.

Personalized treatment plans will probably integrate genetic data, enabling the implementation of precision medicine methodologies that account for the distinct genetic composition of an individual when customizing strategies for managing diabetes.

Conclusion

In summary, the transition to individualized treatment regimens for the management of Type 1 diabetes represents a substantial progression in the field of healthcare. Instances of individuals achieving insulin independence serve as concrete illustrations of the benefits that can be derived from customizing treatment approaches to suit specific requirements. Establishing a conducive way of life, engaging in cooperative efforts with healthcare experts, and imbibing forthcoming technological developments are fundamental tenets within this dynamic framework of diabetes management. Moving forward, the prioritization of customization not only enhances results but also enables individuals diagnosed with Type 1 diabetes to actively manage their health and overall welfare.

9 7 9 8 8 7 6 8 5 0 2 3 2